DASH DIET

The Beginner's Guide to Lose Weight and Lower Blood Pressure (Includes 31-Day Meal Plan)

Ava Young

Copyright@2019

Table of Contents

Introduction

The full meaning of DASH is Dietary Approaches to Stop Hypertension. It is a balanced and flexible eating plan that assists in creating a heart-healthy eating practice for life. There is no requirement for a special food but instead DASH offers weekly and daily nutritional goals. The DASH eating plan recommends:

- Limiting sweets and sugar-sweetened beverages.
- Limiting foods that have high saturated fat. Examples include full-fat dairy products, fatty meats, as well as tropical oils like palm oils, palm kernels, and coconut.
- Incorporating vegetable oils, nuts, beans, poultry, fish, and low-fat or fat-free dairy products.
- Consuming whole grains, fruits, and vegetables.

This book provides information on the DASH diet in order to live healthy, prevent heart disease, reduce blood pressure, and lose weight.

Chapter 1

DASH Diet Versions
The DASH diet recommends that you minimize the amount of sodium you consume. Sodium can increase blood pressure in some people.

The DASH diet have two versions:

- **The standard DASH diet** – this version limits the amount of sodium consumption to a maximum of 2,300 milligrams (mg) per day.

- **The low-sodium DASH diet** – this version restricts the amount of sodium consumption to a maximum of 1,500mg per day.
Both DASH diet versions aim to minimize the sodium levels in your diet as opposed to what you may get in a regular diet, which can be up

to a massive 3,400mg of sodium per day or even more.

The American Heart Association suggests that daily consumption of sodium should be kept at a maximum of 1,500mg per day. The low-sodium DASH diet fulfills this need.

The Dietary Guidelines for Americans recommends that daily consumption of sodium should be kept at a maximum of 2,300mg per day. The standard DASH diet fulfills this need.

If you are unsure of the sodium level that is appropriate for you, discuss this with your doctor.

Chapter 2

Dash Diet Nutrition Basics

Both DASH diet versions include lots of low-fat dairy products, vegetables, fruits, and whole grains. The DASH diet also contains some legumes, poultry and fish, and recommends a small amount of seeds and nuts a few times per week. You can eat fats, sweets and red meat in small quantities.

The DASH diet does not have a lot of total fat, trans-fat and saturated fat.

Based on the 2,000-calorie-a-day DASH diet, below are the recommended servings for each food group.

Legumes, seeds and nuts: *4 to 5 servings per week.*

Lentils, peas, kidney beans, sunflower seeds, almonds and other related foods in this category are good sources of protein, potassium and magnesium.

They're also filled with fiber and phytochemicals – these are plant compounds that might protect against some cardiovascular disease and cancer. Serving sizes are little and are meant to be eaten only a few times per week since these foods have higher calories.

Examples of a single serving include ½ cup cooked peas or beans, 2 tablespoons nut butter or seeds, or 1/3 cup nuts.

- Soybean-based products like tempeh and tofu, can be a good substitute to meat since they contain every amino acid needed by your body to make a full protein, just like meat.

- Nuts are sometimes looked at negatively due to their fat content, however they contain healthy forms of fat — omega-3 fatty acids and monounsaturated fat. Nuts have high calories, so they should be eaten in moderate quantities. Try adding them to cereals, salads or stir-fries.

Dairy: 2 to 3 servings per day.
Cheese, yogurt, milk, and other dairy items are major sources of protein, vitamin D and calcium. But it is essential that you select dairy products that are fat-free or low-fat because if not they can be a huge source of fat — mostly saturated.

Examples of a single serving include 1½ ounces part-skim cheese, 1 cup low-fat yogurt, or 1 cup of skimmed milk/1 percent milk.

- Use regular cheeses and even fat-free cheeses in moderation because they are usually high in sodium.

- If you have difficulty digesting dairy products, select lactose-free products or consider purchasing an over-the-counter product that have the enzyme lactase, which is used to prevent or reduce the signs of lactose intolerance.

- Fat-free or low-fat frozen yogurt can assist you in boosting the quantity of dairy products you consume while providing a sweet treat. You can add fruit to get a healthy twist.

Vegetables: 4 to 5 servings per day.
Greens, sweet potatoes, broccoli, carrots, tomatoes and other vegetables are filled with vitamins, fibers, and such minerals like magnesium and potassium.
Examples of a single serving include ½ cup cooked/ cut-up raw vegetables or 1 cup raw leafy green vegetables.

- To increase the amount of servings you get on a daily basis, be creative. For example, in a stir-fry, reduce the quantity of meat by half and increase the vegetables.

- Frozen and fresh vegetables are both good options. When buying canned and frozen vegetables, select those labeled as low-sodium or with no added salt.
- Don't regard vegetables as only side-dishes — a hearty mix of vegetables served on top of whole-wheat noodles or brown rice can be the main dish.

Sweets: 5 servings or less per week

You do not need to completely remove sweets while on the DASH diet — just don't overindulge.

Examples of a single serving include 1 cup lemonade, ½ cup sorbet, or 1 tablespoon jam, jelly or sugar.

- Reduce the amount of added sugar that doesn't provide any nutritional value but can have a lot of calories.
- Artificial sweeteners such as sucralose (Splenda) and aspartame (Equal,

NutraSweet) may aid in satisfying your sweet tooth while limiting the sugar. But note that you should still use them reasonably. It's OK to exchange a diet soda for a regular soda, but not as a replacement of a more nutritious drink like low-fat milk or even ordinary water.

- When you eat sweets, select those that are low-fat or fat-free, such as low-fat cookies, graham crackers, hard candy, jellybeans, fruit ices, or sorbets.

Fish, poultry and lean meat: *6 one-ounce servings or less per day.*

Meat can be an abundant source of zinc, iron, B vitamins and protein. Choose lean varieties and try for a maximum of 6 one-ounce servings per day. Reducing your meat portion will create room for additional vegetables. Examples of a single serving include 1 ounce of cooked fish, poultry or meat, or 1 egg.

- Eat heart-healthy fish, like tuna, herring and salmon. These kinds of fish have high omega-3 fatty acids that are healthy for the heart.
- Trim away fat and skin from meat and poultry and then roast, grill, broil or bake rather than frying in fat.

Fruits*: about 4 to 5 servings per day.*
Several fruits need minimal preparation in order to be a healthy aspect of a snack or meal. Like vegetables, they're filled with magnesium, potassium and fiber and are usually low in fat — one exception to this is coconut.
Examples of a single serving include 4 ounces of juice, 1/2 cup canned, frozen or fresh fruit, or one medium fruit.
- If you purchase juice or canned, make sure that it doesn't contain added sugar.

- Remember that citrus juices and fruits,
  such as grapefruit, can affect certain
  medications, so discuss with your
  pharmacist or doctor to know if it is
  appropriate.
- Make use of edible peels when possible.
  The peels from fruits such as pears, apples
  and several other fruits puts a nice texture
  to recipes and contain healthy fiber and
  nutrients.
- Eat a piece of fruit during meals and eat
  one as a snack. Afterwards, you can
  complete the day with a dessert made up of
  fresh fruits that is topped with a tablespoon
  of low-fat yogurt.

Grains*: 6 to 8 servings per day*
Grains include pasta, rice, cereal and bread.
Examples of a single serving include ½ cup
cooked pasta, rice or cereal, 1-ounce dry
cereal, or 1 slice whole-wheat bread.

- Focus on whole grains since they have more nutrients and fiber than refined grains do. For example, use whole-grain bread rather than white bread, whole-wheat pasta rather than regular pasta or brown rice rather than white rice. Search for products labeled as "100% whole wheat" or "100% whole grain."
- Grains are low in fat, by nature. Keep them like this by avoiding cheese sauces, cream and butter.

Oils and fats*: 2 to 3 servings per day.*
Fat assists your body in absorbing essential vitamins and assists the immune system of your body. But too much fat raises your risk of obesity, diabetes and heart disease.
The DASH diet pushes for a healthy balance through the restriction of total fat to a maximum of 30% of daily calories gotten from

fat, with an emphasis on the beneficial monounsaturated fats.

Examples of a single serving include 2 tablespoons of salad dressing, 1 tablespoon of mayonnaise or 1 teaspoon of soft margarine.

- Read the food labels on salad dressing and margarine so that you can buy foods that are free of trans-fat and have minimal saturated fat.

- Avoid trans-fat, usually found in processed foods. For example: fried items, baked goods and crackers.

- Trans-fat and saturated fat are the chief dietary culprits in raising the risk of coronary artery related diseases. DASH assists in keeping the daily saturated fat to a maximum of 6% of your whole calories by restricting use of eggs, cream, whole milk, cheese, butter and meat in your diet, as well as foods made from coconut oil, palm oil, solid shortenings and lard.

What Not to Eat

When you are on the DASH plan, you need to limit the amount you eat of the below foods:

- Packaged snacks that are often high in sugar, salt and fat.

- Foods that contain lots of saturated fats, such as deep-fried foods and whole fat dairy.

- Sugar-sweetened beverages. Those that consume fewer calories (individuals not physically active or smaller individuals) should try to totally avoid foods with extra sugar. This might include syrup, jelly and hard candy. Those that consume calories moderately can eat up to five treats a week, and those that are very active may eat less than two per day.

- Alcohol. Adult beverages like spirits, wine, and beer are not completely off-limits, but it is recommended that you limit your consumption. If you consume alcoholic drinks, do within reasonable limits. Drinking moderately can be described as having a maximum of one drink a day for women and a maximum of two drinks a day for men.

- Adding unnecessary salt to food or eating foods with excess salt. Before using salt substitutes (which usually contain potassium) or increasing the level of potassium in your diet, check with your doctor. People that have kidney issues or take certain medicines should be careful about the quantity of potassium they consume.

Chapter 3

Tips for Cooking and Shopping

Staying on the DASH diet begins with the food you purchase. Before going grocery shopping:

- ***Make sure to eat first.*** Do not shop for groceries while you are hungry. If you shop while you are hungry, all food items will look appealing, making it difficult to resist those high-sodium, high-fat items.

- ***Create a list.*** Make a decision regarding the meals you are going to prepare for the upcoming week, and make a note of the ingredients needed. Do not forget to make plans for both snacks and breakfast. Taking this list with you to the store will reduce the likelihood of you being tempted by unhealthy foods.

Bargain prices and large displays may catch your attention when you are in the grocery

store. To remain focused on those foods that
maintain the DASH diet, follow these tips:

- **_Read labels._** Most of the packaged foods
  in the country have a label for "Nutrition
  Facts" that can assist you in figuring out if
  they are the right fit for your diet. Foods
  with low sodium have a maximum of 5%
  for its daily value of sodium per serving.
  Search for reduced fat and sodium
  products. Compare similar items and select
  the one that have lower fat and sodium and
  has fewer calories.

- **_Buy fresh food._** Processed foods contain
  majority of the sodium found in a typical
  diet. Fresh foods are healthier options
  because they have less sodium, along with
  less added fat and sugar. Fresh foods also
  often contain more health-promoting fiber,
  minerals and vitamins than packaged
  foods.

- **Shop the sides.** Even though there are several DASH diet-friendly food ingredients in the center aisles, spend the majority of your shopping time in the outermost aisles where you will find lean meats, low-fat dairy products and fresh produce.

It is more likely for you to prepare healthy dishes when you already have healthy food options on hand. Try to store these items in the kitchen:

- **Spreads, seasonings and condiments.** Olive oil, salsas, flavored vinegars, spices and herbs can add flavor to your meals with no salt overload. Select reduced or low sodium versions of condiments.
- **Fish, poultry and lean meats.** Choose lean selections, like sirloin or round beef cuts, extra-lean ground beef, pork

tenderloin, skinless turkey, skinless chicken, and fish. Look for poultry that is not injected with broth or fat. Choose lower sodium canned meat and fish. Limit processed or smoked meats, like deli meats.

- ***Legumes, seeds and nuts.*** Sunflower seeds, chickpeas (garbanzos), lentils, kidney beans, walnuts and almonds are among the healthy choices. But get low-salt or unsalted varieties.
- ***Grains.*** Purchase whole-grain varieties of tortillas, crackers, pasta, rice, cereal, pitas, bagels and bread. Compare labels and select lower sodium items.
- ***Low-fat dairy products.*** Search for reduced fat dairy options when purchasing sour cream, yogurt, cheeses, buttermilk and milk.
- ***Vegetables.*** Buy canned, frozen or fresh vegetables, such as spinach, broccoli, carrots and tomatoes. Select frozen

vegetables with no added sauces or butter or salt. Go for canned vegetables that are low in sodium.

- ***Fruits.*** Choose an assortment of fresh fruits, like bananas, oranges and apples. Add variety with berries, dates and apricots. Select frozen fruits with no added sugar and fruit that is canned in its own juice (instead of heavy syrup).

Your kitchen gadgets and cookware can make it simpler to maintain the DASH diet. Useful items include:

- ***Garlic press or spice mill.*** These items make it simple to add spices to your food and minimize your reliance on the saltshaker.

- ***Vegetable steamer.*** This fits into the bottom of a pot. It makes it easy to cook vegetables without losing any nutrient and with no added fat and calories.

- ***Nonstick cookware.*** This reduces the
  need to make use of butter or oil when
  sautéing vegetables or meat.

Cooking habits that are unhealthy can destroy
your other efforts to keep to the DASH diet.
Make use of these tips to assist in reducing fat
and sodium:

- ***Cut back on meat.*** Cook casseroles and
  stews with about two-thirds of the meat
  called for by the recipe, and add extra
  whole-wheat pasta, bulgur, tofu, brown rice
  or vegetables.
- ***Make lower fat substitutions.*** Exchange full-fat dairy
  with fat-free or reduced-fat versions.
- ***Be cautious of broth.*** You can prepare
  onions, mushrooms, or any other vegetable
  in a small low-sodium broth within a
  nonstick pan. A small amount of healthy oil
  (like olive oil) may be a better choice, since

even low-sodium broth can contain lots of sodium.

- **_Rinse well._** Canned foods such as vegetables and beans, should be rinsed before usage to wash away some extra salt.

- **_Spice it up._** Improve flavor without adding fat or salt by using sodium-free bouillon, garlic powder or garlic, lemon, ginger, peppers, onions, flavored vinegars, spices or herbs.

If you usually bake or cook in ways that require lots of salt and fat, don't be afraid to change your recipes. Experiment with substitutions and spices. Diversify and attempt recipes you would not usually try. You might come to discover new delicious ways to prepare your favorite recipes.

Chapter 4

Recommendations

Try these approaches to start your DASH diet
journey:

- ***Get support when needed***. If it is
  getting hard for you to stick to your diet,
  discuss this with your dietitian or doctor.
  You might get some suggestions that will
  aid you in continuing with the DASH diet.

- ***Add physical activity.*** To improve your
  blood pressure and weight loss goals,
  consider raising your physical activity while
  following the DASH diet. Merging both the
  physical activity and DASH diet makes it
  more possible to reduce your blood
  pressure and reach your weight loss goal.

- ***Forgive slip-ups and reward
  successes***. Reward yourself for your
  accomplishments with a nonfood treat —
  hangout with a friend, purchase a book, or

rent a movie. Everyone falters, especially when discovering something new. Bear in mind that altering your lifestyle is a lengthy process. Find out what led to your setback in the first place, and then continue from where you stopped with the DASH diet.

- **_Change slowly_**. If currently, you eat just one or a couple servings of vegetables or fruits per day, try to add one serving at lunch and another at dinner. Instead of completely switching to whole grains, begin by having one or two servings of whole grains. Gradually increasing your intake of whole grains, vegetables and fruits can also assist in preventing diarrhea or bloating that may take place if you are not used to having a diet with plenty fiber. You can also attempt to take over-the-counter products to aid in reducing gas from vegetables and beans.

Handling Slip-ups and Barriers

Take the time to figure out the things that could negatively affect your DASH diet journey. These are known as barriers. And by examining them now, you can make plans on how to handle them when they occur. A good example of a barrier may involve eating in restaurants. If this is something you do a lot, you might have to make plans on how you will remain on your DASH diet while eating out. Possible solutions include:

- Find restaurants that provide low-fat and vegetarian dishes.
- Look at menus in advance to find meals you can consume and still remain on your eating plan.
- Eat out less often.

It's perfectly normal to attempt something, stop midway, and then get angry at yourself.

Several people have to try over and over again before they achieve their goals.

- Don't forget small rewards. Something to anticipate can keep you going.

- When you encounter a barrier—and several people do—get support. Reach out to your friends and family members to see if anyone wants to cheer you on or go on this journey with you.

- If you feel like quitting, don't waste energy berating yourself. Remember your purpose for wanting to change, reflect on your progress so far, and encourage yourself. Then you may want to try again.

Getting Support

Having a large amount of support can simplify the process of changing your eating habits. For instance, if family members let you know that they like how you are getting and looking healthier, you may be encouraged to continue. Here are some other means to get support:

- ***Don't forget to give yourself a reward.*** When you reach a milestone or accomplish one of your goals, reward yourself with a gift. Do everything it takes just to remind yourself that you have been achieving your goals.

- ***Join a support group or class.*** People in these groups usually encountered some of the barriers you are experiencing.

- ***Family members and friends*** can eat healthy foods with you. They can motivate you by letting you know how they respect you for making difficult changes.

- ***Work with a partner.*** It's encouraging to know that someone else has the same goals as you do.

Chapter 5

31-Day Dash Diet Meal Plan

Heart-Healthy Tip: Do not put the additional pinch of salt to assist in keeping the sodium below the recommended levels.

Day 1

Breakfast

Yogurt with raspberries and nuts. (251 calories)

- 1 tsp. honey.
- 5 walnuts, chopped.
- ½ cup raspberries.
- 1 cup of nonfat plain Greek yogurt.

Top yogurt with honey, walnuts and raspberries.

Morning snack

Cinnamon apple. (95 calories)

- Ground cinnamon to taste.
- 1 medium apple, sliced.

Sprinkle apple slices with the grinded cinnamon.

Lunch

- 1 serving of avocado and white bean toast.
- 1 tbsp. of all-purpose vinaigrette.
- 2 tbsp. of grated carrot.
- ½ cup cucumber slices.
- 1½ cups mixed greens.

Top salad greens with vinaigrette, carrot, and cucumber. Toss to combine. (332 calories)

Afternoon snack

- 1 medium plum. (30 calories)

Dinner

- Hummus dressing on 1 serving of stuffed sweet potato. (472 calories)

Daily totals: 976mg sodium, 36g fat, 46g fiber, 176g carbohydrates, 58g protein, 1,180 calories.

Day 2

Breakfast

Honey and fig yogurt. (258 calories)

- 1½ tsp. honey.

- 2 tsp. chia seeds.

- 5 dried figs, chopped.

- 2/3 cup of nonfat plain Greek yogurt.

Top yogurt with honey, chia seeds, and figs.

Morning snack

- 1 cup raspberries. (64 calories)

Lunch

Pear and turkey pita melt. (342 calories)

- 1 cup mixed greens.

- 1 tbsp. of shredded Cheddar cheese.

- 1 medium sliced pear.

- 3½ oz. of low-sodium deli turkey.

- ½ of a large round whole-wheat pita.

Stuff the pita with cheese, ½ of the pear slices, and turkey. Toast inside a toaster oven till the cheese begins to melt. Add greens onto the pita right before eating. Place the other pear slices at the side.

Afternoon snack (83 calories)

- 4 walnuts halves.
- 1 medium plum.

Dinner (469 calories)

- 1 clementine and 1 serving of chocolate bites, to snack on after dinner.
- 1 serving of lemon-garlic shrimp onto Orzo with Zucchini added.

Daily totals: 1,290mg sodium, 31g fat, 30g fiber, 162g carbohydrates, 80g protein, 1,216 calories.

Day 3

Breakfast

Egg toast with salsa. (266 calories)

- 2 tbsp. salsa.

- A pinch of salt and a pinch of pepper.

- 1 egg, cooked with 1/4 tsp. olive oil.

- 1 slice of whole-wheat bread, toasted.

Top bread with salsa, pepper, salt and egg.

- 1 medium banana.

Morning snack (136 calories)

- 2 tbsp. hummus.

- ½ large whole-wheat round pita, toasted.

Lunch

- 1½ cups of chicken chili together with sweet potatoes. (324 calories)

Afternoon snack

- ½ cup raspberries. (32 calories)

Dinner (448 calories)

- ½ ounce of dark chocolate, to snack on after dinner.
- 1 1/3 cups of creamy fettuccine together with mushrooms and brussels sprouts.

Daily totals: 1,754mg sodium, 36g fat, 30g fiber, 171g carbohydrates, 62g protein, 1,206 calories.

Day 4

Breakfast

- 1 serving of peanut-butter cinnamon toast. (266 calories)

Morning snack

- 1 cup raspberries. (64 calories)

Lunch (342 calories)

- 1 cup grapes.

- 1 serving of salmon pita sandwich.

Afternoon snack

Cinnamon pears (102 calories)

- Grinded cinnamon to add taste.

- 1 sliced medium pear.

Sprinkle the ground cinnamon on the pear slices.

Dinner (437 calories)

- 1 clementine, to snack on after dinner.

- Orzo salad with 1 serving of Mediterranean chicken.

Daily totals: 1,234mg sodium, 35g fat, 30 g fiber, 164g carbohydrates, 69g protein, 1,211 calories.

Day 5

Breakfast (355 calories)

- 1 cup blueberries.

- 1 serving of avocado egg toast.

Morning snack

- 1 cup strawberries. (46 calories)

Lunch (372 calories)

- 1 slice of whole-wheat bread, toasted.
- 1 serving of tuna, white bean and dill salad.

Afternoon snack

- 1 medium orange. (62 calories)

Dinner

- 1 serving of kale, potatoes, and skillet lemon chicken. (374 calories)

Daily Totals: 1,289mg sodium, 9g saturated fat, 50g fat, 27g fiber, 130g carbohydrates, 64g protein, 1,209 calories.

Day 6

Breakfast (328 calories)

- 1 cup of blueberries.

- 1 cup of skim milk.

- 1 cup of bran cereal.

Morning snack

- 1 medium orange. (62 calories)

Lunch

- 1 serving of tuna, white bean and dill salad. (296 calories)

Afternoon snack

- 1 cup strawberries. (46 calories)

Dinner

- 1 serving of toaster-oven tostada. (457 calories)

Daily totals: 1,203mg sodium, 8g saturated fat, 39g fat, 49g fiber, 184g carbohydrates, 55g protein, 1,189 calories.

Day 7

Breakfast (293 calories)

- ½ cup sliced strawberries.
- ½ cup of rolled oats, boiled in 1 cup milk. Cook oats and add a pinch of cinnamon and top with strawberries.

Morning snack (90 calories)

- 3 tbsp. hummus.
- ½ bell pepper, sliced.

Lunch

- 1 serving of loaded black-bean nacho soup. (350 calories)

Afternoon snack

- 1 cup blueberries. (84 calories)

Dinner

- 1¼ cups of chicken cauliflower fried "rice". (304 calories)

Evening snack

- ¾ cup kiwi and mango with fresh lime zest. (92 calories)

Daily totals: 1,170mg sodium, 8g saturated fat, 42g fat, 31g fiber, 161g carbohydrates, 62g protein, 1,213 calories.

Day 8

Breakfast (265 calories)

- ½ cup blueberries.
- ¾ cup skim milk.
- 1 cup bran cereal.

Morning snack

- 1 medium apple. (95 calories)

Lunch (374 calories)

- 1 serving of green salad with hummus and pita bread.

Afternoon snack

- 1 medium orange. (62 calories)

Dinner (407 calories)

- 1 cup of steamed broccoli mixed with 1 tsp. of olive oil.
- ½ cup of cooked brown rice.
- 1 serving of Cod and tomato cream sauce.

Daily Totals: 1,370mg sodium, 8g saturated fat, 34g fat, 43g fiber, 195g carbohydrates, 54g protein, 1,203 calories.

Day 9

Breakfast (276 calories)

- 2 tsp. honey.

- 1½ tbsp. of slivered almonds.
- ½ cup blueberries.
- 1 cup of nonfat plain Greek yogurt.

Top yogurt with honey, almonds and blueberries.

Morning snack (102 calories)

- 2 tbsp. hummus.
- 2 medium carrots.

Lunch (320 calories)

- 1½ cups of peanut noodle salad and roasted tofu.

Afternoon snack

- 1 cup strawberries. (46 calories)

Dinner (460 calories)

- 1 cup of cooked quinoa mixed with 1 tsp. of olive oil plus a pinch of salt.

- 1 serving of paprika-herb rubbed chicken.
- 1 serving of grilled romaine plus an avocado-lime dressing.

Daily totals: 1,263mg sodium, 6g saturated fat, 42g fat, 26g fiber, 135g carbohydrates, 79g protein, 1,204 calories.

Day 10

Breakfast (287 calories)

- ½ cup blueberries.
- 1 cup skim milk.
- 1 cup bran cereal.

Morning snack

- 1 medium apple. (95 calories)

Lunch

- 1 serving of veggie-hummus sandwich. (325 calories)

Afternoon snack (80 calories)

- 2 tbsp. hummus.
- ¾ sliced medium red bell pepper.

Dinner (426 calories)

- 2 cups of peanut noodle salad and roasted tofu.

Daily totals: 1,324mg sodium, 6g saturated fat, 42g fat, 48g fiber, 183g carbohydrates, 55g protein, 1,213 calories.

Day 11

Breakfast (367 calories)

- 1 tbsp. of slivered almonds.
- 1 cup blueberries.
- 1 cup bran cereal.
- 1 cup nonfat milk.

Top cereal with slivered almonds and blueberries.

Morning snack (266 calories)

- ¼ cup raisins.

- 2 tbsp. walnuts.

- 1 medium orange.

Lunch (461 calories)

- 1 medium apple.

- 1 slice of whole-wheat bread, halved.

- 1 serving of tuna, white bean and dill salad.

Afternoon snack (234 calories)

- 1 tbsp. chia seeds.

- 1 cup of plain nonfat yogurt.

- 1 cup strawberries.

Top yogurt with chia seeds and strawberries.

Dinner

- 1 serving of toaster-oven tostada. (457 calories)

Evening snack (219 calories)

- 3 cups of air-popped popcorn mixed with 1 tbsp. each of no-salt-added herb seasoning/garlic and olive oil.

Daily totals: 1,529mg sodium, 4,945mg potassium, 12g saturated fat, 72g fat, 66g fiber, 295g carbohydrate, 83g protein, 2,004 calories.

Day 12

Breakfast (451 calories)

- 1 medium banana.
- 2 tbsp. chopped walnuts.
- 1 serving of quick-cooking oats.

Top oats with a pinch of cinnamon, banana, and walnuts.

Morning snack (330 calories)

- 1 tbsp. chia seeds.
- 1½ cup of plain nonfat yogurt.

- 1 cup of thawed frozen raspberries.

Top yogurt with chia seeds, almonds and raspberries.

Lunch (416 calories)

- 1 serving of quick creamy tomato Cup-of-Soup.

Easy Grilled Cheese

- 3 tbsp. of shredded Cheddar cheese.
- 2 slices of whole-wheat bread.
- 2 tsp. olive oil.

Heat oil in skillet. Put a slice of bread in the heated skillet. Place cheese on top as well as the remaining slice of bread. Heat on both sides until the cheese melts and it becomes golden brown.

Afternoon snack (318 calories)

- ¼ cup raisins.
- 1 tbsp. peanut butter.
- 1 medium banana.

Dinner (399 calories)

- 2 cups of mixed greens tossed with 2 tsp. vinegar and 1 tbsp. olive oil.
- 1 serving of herbed baked potatoes and sour cream.

Evening Snack

- 2 servings of strawberry ice cream. (179 calories)

Daily Totals: 1,281mg sodium, 5,736 mg potassium, 16g saturated fat, 69g fat, 46g fiber, 299g carbohydrate, 67g protein, 2,093 calories.

Day 13

Breakfast (419 calories)

- 1 medium orange.
- 1 serving of spinach-avocado smoothie.

Morning snack (218 calories)

- 1½ tbsp. of chia seeds.
- ½ cup of plain nonfat yogurt.
- 1 cup of thawed frozen raspberries.

Top yogurt with chia seeds, walnuts and raspberries.

Lunch (491 calories)

- 1 medium apple.
- 1 serving of quick turkey Bolognese and zucchini noodles mixed with 1 1/2 tbsp. olive oil infused with basil.

Afternoon snack

- ¼ cup almonds. (206 calories)

Dinner (431 calories)

- 1 cup of mixed greens tossed with 1 tsp. vinegar and 2 tsp. olive oil.
- 1 serving barley and bean soup.

Evening snack (219 calories)

- 3 cups of air-popped popcorn mixed with 1 tbsp. each of no-salt-added herb seasoning/garlic and olive oil.

Daily totals: 1,530mg sodium, 4,763mg potassium, 15g saturated fat, 109g fat, 54g fiber, 230g carbohydrate, 73g protein, 1,984 calories.

Day 14

Breakfast (419 calories)

- 1 medium orange.
- 1 serving of spinach-avocado smoothie.

Morning snack (219 calories)

- 3 tbsp. almonds.
- 1 cup raspberries.

Lunch (491 calories)

- 1 medium apple.
- 1 serving of quick turkey Bolognese and zucchini noodles mixed with 1 1/2 tbsp. olive oil infused with basil.

Afternoon snack (210 calories)

- 1 tbsp. peanut butter.
- 1 medium banana.

Dinner (506 calories)

- 5-oz. glass red wine.
- 1 serving of southwestern salmon cobb salad.

Evening snack (177 calories)

- 3 cups of air-popped popcorn mixed with 1 tbsp. each of no-salt-added herb seasoning/garlic and olive oil.

Daily totals: 1,527mg sodium, 5,365mg potassium, 20g saturated fat, 95g fat, 44g fiber, 199g carbohydrate, 90g protein, 2,022 calories.

Day 15

Breakfast (419 calories)

- 1 medium orange.
- 1 serving of spinach-avocado smoothie.

Morning snack (133 calories)

- 6 walnut halves.
- 1 cup cubed cantaloupe.

Lunch (431 calories)

- 1 medium apple.
- 1 serving of quick turkey Bolognese and zucchini noodles mixed with 1½ tbsp. olive oil infused with basil.

Afternoon snack (263 calories)

- 1½ tbsp. of peanut butter.

- 1 medium banana.

Dinner (528 calories)

- 1 tbsp. of slivered almonds to place on the salad.
- 1 serving of green salad and vinaigrette.
- 1 serving of kale, potatoes, and lemon chicken.

Evening snack (201 calories)

- ¼ cup raisins
- 3 cups of air-popped popcorn mixed with 1 tbsp. each of no-salt-added herb seasoning/garlic and olive oil.

Daily totals: 1,473mg sodium, 5,176mg potassium, 15.5g saturated fat, 88g fat, 37g fiber, 238g carbohydrate, 80g protein, 1,975 calories.

Day 16

Breakfast (380 calories)

- 1 medium orange.
- 1 serving of strawberry-banana green smoothie.

Morning snack (235 calories)

- 1 tbsp. chia seeds.
- 2 tsp. honey.
- ½ cup of plain nonfat yogurt.
- 1 cup of thawed frozen raspberries.

Top yogurt with chia seeds, honey and raspberries.

Lunch (501 calories)

- 1 tbsp. peanut butter.
- 1 medium apple, sliced.
- 1 serving of quick turkey Bolognese and zucchini noodles mixed with 1 1/2 tbsp. olive oil infused with basil.

Afternoon snack (159 calories)

- 8 walnut halves.

- 1 cup of cubed cantaloupe.

Dinner (526 calories)

- 1 tbsp. of slivered almonds to place on top of salad.

- ½ serving of green Salad and vinaigrette.

- 1 serving of easy spinach and pea carbonara.

Evening snack

- 2 servings of strawberry ice Cream. (179 calories)

Daily Totals: 1,528mg sodium, 4,778mg potassium, 15g saturated fat, 77g fat, 53g fiber, 265g carbohydrate, 82g protein, 1,980 calories.

Day 17

Breakfast (437 calories)

- ½ serving of spinach-avocado smoothie.
- ¼ cup raisins.
- 1 serving of quick-cooking oats.

Top oats with a pinch of cinnamon and raisins. Enjoy with half of the smoothie.

Morning snack (243 calories)

- 1 cup raspberries.
- ½ serving of spinach-avocado smoothie.

Lunch (400 calories)

- 1 serving of quick creamy tomato Cup-of-Soup.

Easy Grilled Cheese

- 3 tbsp. of shredded Cheddar cheese.
- 2 slices of whole-wheat bread.
- 2 tsp. unsalted butter.

Spread butter on both sides of the bread slices. Put a slice, buttered-side down, onto a heated skillet. Put cheese on top and butter the order slice. Cook on both sides until the cheese melts and it turns golden brown.

Afternoon snack (210 calories)

- 1 tbsp. peanut butter.
- 1 medium banana.

Dinner (577 calories)

- 1½ cup of easy brown rice.
- 1 serving of pineapple slaw and jerk chicken.

Evening snack

- 2 servings of pineapple ice cream. (109 calories)

Daily totals: 1,454mg sodium, 4,715mg potassium, 15.5g saturated fat, 50g fat, 41g fiber, 319g carbohydrate, 82g protein, 1,976 calories.

Day 18

Breakfast (271 calories)

- 1 serving of avocado egg toast.

Morning snack

- ½ cup blueberries. (42 calories)

Lunch

- 1 serving of Green Salad together with hummus and pita bread. (374 calories)

Afternoon snack

- 1 medium orange. (62 calories)

Dinner (457 calories)

- 1 medium red potato that is baked and spiced using a pinch of pepper, 1 tbsp. of plain nonfat Greek yogurt and 1 tsp. of olive oil.

- 1 cup of steamed green beans.
- 1 serving of seared salmon plus green peppercorn sauce.

Daily totals: 1,296mg sodium, 10 saturated fat, 49g fat, 28g fiber, 140g carbohydrates, 62g protein, 1,206 calories.

Day 19

Breakfast (266 calories)

Egg toast with salsa

- 2 tbsp. of salsa.
- Pinch each of pepper and salt.
- 1 egg, boiled in ¼ tsp. of olive oil.
- 1 slice of toasted whole-wheat bread.

Top bread with the salsa, pepper, salt and egg.

- 1 medium banana.

Morning snack

Cinnamon pears

- Ground cinnamon to taste.

- 1 pear, sliced.

Sprinkle cinnamon on the pear slices. (102 calories)

Lunch (325 calories)

- 1 serving of veggie-hummus sandwich.

Afternoon snack

- ¾ cup raspberries. (48 calories)

Dinner (450 calories)

- 1 serving of lemon-herb spiced salmon together with Farro Caponata.

Daily Totals: 1,438mg sodium, 40g fat, 37g fiber, 161g carbohydrates, 60g protein, 1,191 calories.

Day 20

Breakfast (266 calories)

- 1 serving of peanut-butter cinnamon toast.

Morning snack

- 2 clementine. (70 calories)

Lunch

Green salad with hummus and pita bread.
(332 calories)

- ¼ cup hummus.
- ½ large whole-wheat round pita.
- 2 tbsp. of all-purpose vinaigrette.
- ½ cup of sliced cucumber.
- ¼ cup of grated carrot.
- 2 cups mixed greens.

Top greens with vinaigrette, cucumber and
carrot. Serve with hummus and pita bread.

Afternoon snack (104 calories)

- 1 medium plum.
- 1 cup grapes.

Dinner (412 calories)

- 1 tbsp. of nonfat plain Greek yogurt.

- ¼ avocado, diced.

- 1½ cups of chicken chili together with sweet potatoes.

Top chili with yogurt and avocado.

Daily Totals: 1,322mg sodium, 42g fat, 31g fiber, 166g carbohydrates, 50g protein, 1,184 calories.

Day 21

Breakfast

Honey and fig yogurt. (258 calories)

- 1½ tsp. honey.

- 2 tsp. chia seeds.

- 5 dried figs, chopped.

- 2/3 cup of nonfat plain Greek yogurt.

Top yogurt with honey, chia seeds, and figs.

Morning snack

- ½ cup grapes. (52 calories)

Lunch

Avocado and white bean salad. (350 calories)

- 2 tbsp. of all-purpose vinaigrette.
- ½ avocado, diced.
- 1/3 cup of canned white beans, rinsed.
- ¾ cup chopped veggies, like cherry tomatoes and cucumbers.
- 2 cups mixed greens.

Top salad greens with vinaigrette, avocado, beans and veggies. Toss to combine.

Afternoon snack

- 1 clementine. (35 calories)

Dinner (489 calories)

- 1 serving of chocolate bites, to snack on after dinner.

- 1 serving of curried cauliflower steaks plus tzatziki and red rice.

Daily Totals: 818mg sodium, 53g fat, 30g fiber, 155g carbohydrates, 41g protein, 1,184 calories.

Day 22

Breakfast (268 calories)

- 2 tbsp. maple granola.
- 1 medium peach, chopped.
- 1 cup of low-fat plain Greek yogurt.

Top yogurt with granola and peach.

Morning snack

- 1 cup raspberries. (64 calories)

Lunch

- 11 serving of chicken satay bowls plus spicy peanut sauce. (351 calories)

Afternoon snack

- ½ cup blackberries. (31 calories)

Dinner (454 calories)

- 1½ cups of massaged kale salad.

- 1 serving of lemon-pepper linguine with squash.

Dessert

- 1 serving of berry-lemon ice pops. (53 calories)

Daily Totals: 1,220mg sodium, 52g fat, 29g fiber, 141g carbohydrates, 61g protein, 1,221 calories.

Day 23

Breakfast

- 1 serving of pineapple green smoothie. (297 calories)

Morning snack

- ½ cup raspberries. (32 calories)

Lunch

- 1 serving of chicken satay bowls together with spicy peanut sauce. (351 calories)

Afternoon snack (4 calories)

- ¼ cup of sliced cucumber topped with one pinch of pepper and salt.

Dinner (488 calories)

- 1 serving of guacamole chopped salad.
- 1 serving of southwest flank steak together with fresh tomatillo salsa.

Dessert

- 1 serving of berry-lemon ice pops. (53 calories)

Daily Totals: 1,205mg sodium, 59g fat, 29g fiber, 108g carbohydrates, 76g protein, 1,225 calories.

Day 24

Breakfast

- 1 serving of pineapple green smoothie. (297 calories)

Morning snack

- 1 small peach. (51 calories)

Lunch

- 1 serving of vegetarian niçoise salad. (366 calories)

Afternoon snack

- ½ cup blackberries. (31 calories)

Dinner (473 calories)

- 1 serving avocado pineapple salad.
- 1 serving of grilled blackened shrimp tacos.

Daily Totals: 1,314mg sodium, 53g fat, 33g fiber, 146g carbohydrates, 53g protein, 1,218 calories,

Day 25

Breakfast

Tomato and egg tortilla. (255 calories)

- 5 cherry tomatoes, halved.
- 1 large egg, fried in 1/4 tsp. of olive oil or spray pan with a tiny layer of cooking spray. Add a pinch of pepper.
- 1 corn tortilla.

Top tortilla with tomatoes and egg.

- 1 medium banana.

Morning snack

- 2 cups cubed cantaloupe. (109 calories)

Lunch (324 calories)

- 1½ cups of sweet potatoes and chicken chili.

Afternoon snack

- 1 cup strawberries. (46 calories)

Dinner (446 calories)

- ¼ cup grated carrot.

- 2 cups mixed greens.

- 1 serving of stuffed delicata squash.

Top greens with grated carrot and drizzle with 2 tsp. olive oil and 1 tbsp. balsamic vinegar.

Day 26

Breakfast

Banana oatmeal. (266 calories)

- 1 medium banana, sliced.

- 1/3 cup of rolled oats, cooked with 2/3 cup milk.

Cook oats, add a pinch of cinnamon and top with banana.

Morning snack (136 calories)

- 1 tbsp. of unsalted dry-roasted almonds.

- 1 cup blueberries.

Lunch

White bean and tuna salad. (308 calories)

- 2 cups mixed greens.

- 2 tsp. olive oil.

- 1 tbsp. red-wine vinegar.

- ½ cucumber, sliced.

- 8 cherry tomatoes, halved.

- 2½ oz. of chunk light tuna, drained.

- ½ cup of canned white beans, rinsed.

Combine cucumber, tomatoes, tuna, and beans. Toss with oil, vinegar and add a pinch each of pepper and kosher salt. Serve over greens.

Afternoon snack

- 1 medium orange. (62 calories)

Dinner (440 calories)

- 2 cups of mixed greens, add a pinch each of pepper and kosher salt, top with 2 tsp. olive oil. and 1 tbsp. balsamic vinegar

- 1½ cups of sweet potatoes and chicken chili.

Day 27

Breakfast (288 calories)

Almond and blueberry yoghurt parfait.

- 1½ tbsp. of slivered almonds.
- ¼ cup blueberries.
- ¾ cup of nonfat plain Greek yogurt.

Top yogurt with almonds and blueberries.

- 2 cups cubed cantaloupe.

Morning snack

- ½ bell pepper, sliced. (13 calories)

Lunch

Toaster-oven tostadas. (336 calories)

- 2 tbsp. of shredded Cheddar cheese.
- ½ bell pepper, sliced.
- ½ cup corn.
- ½ cup of canned black beans, rinsed.

- 2 corn tortillas.

Top tortillas cheese, bell pepper, corn, and beans. Toast until the cheese starts to melt.

Afternoon snack

- ½ cup blueberries. (42 calories)

Dinner (428 calories)

- 1 diagonal slice of baguette (about 1/4 inch thick), ideally whole-wheat, toasted.
- 2½ cups of shrimp and avocado chopped salad.

Evening snack

- 2 kiwis. (84 calories)

Day 28

Breakfast

Avocado and white bean toast. (270 calories)

- ¼ cup of canned white beans, cleaned and mashed.

- ½ avocado, mashed.
- 1 slice of toasted whole-wheat bread.

Top toast with white beans and mashed avocado. Season with crushed red pepper and a pinch each of pepper and kosher salt.

Morning snack

- 2 medium carrots. (50 calories)

Lunch

Green salad and chicken. (341 calories)

- 2/3 cup of roasted beet salad.
- 3oz. cooked chicken breast.
- 2 cups mixed greens.

Mix ingredients and add 2 tsp. each olive oil and lemon juice.

Afternoon snack

- 1 medium orange. (62 calories)

Dinner (472 calories)

Corn and black bean tacos.

- ¼ cup salsa.

- ½ avocado, diced.

- ½ cup corn.

- ¼ cup of canned black beans, cleaned and
  mashed.

- 2 corn tortillas, warmed.

Spread the beans on tortillas. Top with salsa,
avocado and corn.

- 2 cups of mixed greens. Add a pinch each of
  pepper and kosher salt and topped with 2
  tsp. olive oil, 1 tbsp. lime juice.

Day 29

Breakfast

Almond and blueberry yoghurt parfait. (270
calories)

- 1½ tbsp. of slivered almonds.

- ¼ cup blueberries.

- ¾ cup of nonfat plain Greek yogurt.

Top yogurt with almonds and blueberries.

- 1 2/3 cups of cubed cantaloupe.

Morning snack

- 2 medium carrots. (50 calories)

Lunch

Mixed greens with sliced apple and lentils.
(347 calories)

- 1½ tbsp. of crumbled feta cheese.
- 1 apple, sliced.
- ½ cup cooked lentils.
- 1½ cups mixed greens.

Top greens with feta, ½ apple slices and
lentils. Dress the salad with 2 tsp. olive oil and
1 tbsp. red-wine vinegar. Serve the other half
of the apple slices at the side.

Afternoon snack

- 1 medium orange. (62 calories)

Dinner (448 calories)

- 4oz. chicken breast that is seasoned with a pinch each of pepper and kosher salt and ¼ tsp. cumin and cooked in 1 tsp. of olive oil.
- 1 1/3 cups of roasted beet salad.

Day 30

Breakfast

Strawberry oatmeal. (268 calories)

- ½ cup sliced strawberries.
- ½ cup rolled oats, boiled in 1 cup skim milk.

Cook oats and add a pinch of cinnamon and strawberries.

Morning snack

- 2 cups cubed cantaloupe. (109 calories)

Lunch

Veggie-hummus sandwich. (318 calories)

- 1 cup mixed greens.

- ¼ cup cucumber slices.
- ¼ sliced medium red bell pepper.
- ¼ avocado, mashed.
- 3 tbsp. hummus.
- 2 slices of whole-wheat bread.

Spread avocado and hummus on each slice of bread. Top a slice with vegetables and place the slices together for the sandwich.

Afternoon snack

- 2 medium carrots. (50 calories)

Dinner (472 calories)

- 1 diagonal slice of baguette (about ¼ inch thick), ideally whole-wheat, toasted and top with 2 tbsp. of grated parmesan cheese.
- 1 serving of spaghetti squash with almond pesto, beans, and roasted tomatoes.

Day 31

Breakfast (266 calories)

Egg toast with salsa

- 2 tbsp. salsa.

- A pinch of salt and a pinch of pepper.

- 1 egg, cooked with ¼ tsp. olive oil.

- 1 slice of whole-wheat bread, toasted.

Top toast with salsa and egg.

- 1 medium banana.

Morning snack

- ¾ cup blueberries. (63 calories)

Lunch

Veggie and white beans salad. (343 calories)

- ½ avocado, diced.

- 1/3 cup of white beans, rinsed.

- ¾ cup of your chosen veggies (try tomatoes and cucumbers).

- 2 cups mixed greens.

Mix ingredients and add freshly ground pepper, 2 tsp. olive oil, and 1 tbsp. red-wine vinegar.

Afternoon snack

- 1 medium orange. (62 calories)

Dinner (449 calories)

- ½ cup of cooked lentils that is seasoned with one pinch each of pepper and kosher salt.

- 1 serving of salmon that is roasted and spiced with brussels sprouts and garlic.

Chapter 6

Conclusion

The DASH diet is a balanced and flexible eating plan that assists in creating a heart-healthy eating practice for life. The DASH diet versions include the low-sodium DASH diet and the standard DASH diet. The foods covered by the DASH diet include legumes, seeds and nuts; dairy; vegetables; sweets; fish, poultry and lean meat; fruits; grains; oils and fats. Recommendations to properly implement DASH diet involve getting support when needed, adding physical activity, forgiving slip-ups and rewarding successes, and changing slowly. A 31-day DASH diet meal plan have also been discussed.

www.ingramcontent.com/pod-product-compliance
Lightning Source LLC
Chambersburg PA
CBHW051221250726

48655CB00006B/2526